The Ultimate Guide To Isometric Exercises

A Complete Manual For Senior Fitness: Bodyweight And Isometric Exercises For Enhanced Strength, Balance, And Flexibility In A Simple And Effective Guide

Michael Kessler

Table of Contents

CHAPTER ONE 3
- Isometric Exercises 3
- Isometric Exercises by Muscle Group (Upper Body) 5
- Lower Body 7
- Core 10

CHAPTER TWO 13
- Dynamic Isometric Exercises 13
- Isometric Exercises with Props and Equipment 19
- Advanced isometric training challenging exercises 21

CHAPTER THREE 23
- Isometric Yoga Poses 23
- Creating a Balanced Isometric Workout 24
- Sample Isometric Workout Plan 25
- Isometric training for specific goals 29
- Safety Guidelines and Tips 31
- Conclusion 34

THE END 35

CHAPTER ONE

Isometric Exercises

Isometric exercises are movements where your muscles contract without changing their length, meaning there's no visible movement or joint angle change. Instead, you exert force against an immovable object or resist an opposing force.

The science behind isometric training lies in the muscle contraction itself. When you engage in isometric exercises, the muscle contracts, generating tension without causing the muscle to visibly lengthen or shorten.

This static contraction recruits muscle fibers, enhancing strength and endurance.

Benefits of isometric workouts are varied. They're excellent for building strength in specific joint angles and can help improve stability and endurance. They're low-impact, reducing joint stress, and can be done almost anywhere without the need for equipment.

Isometric Exercises by Muscle Group (Upper Body)

Isometric exercises for the upper body can effectively target various muscle groups. Here are a few examples:

Isometric Push-Up Hold:

- Start in a push-up position.
- Lower yourself until your elbows are at a 90-degree angle.
- Hold this position without moving for a specific duration, engaging your chest, shoulders, and triceps.

Chest Press Hold:

- Sit or stand with your back against a wall.
- Hold your arms at a 90-degree angle, as if you're about to push something away.
- Push your hands against an immovable object or simply press your palms together with force, engaging your chest muscles.

Isometric Shoulder Press:

- Stand or sit with a straight back.
- Hold weights or resistance bands at shoulder height.

- Push up against the weights or bands, holding the position without lifting or lowering them, engaging your shoulder muscles.

Lower Body

Some isometric exercises targeting the lower body:

Isometric Squat Hold:

- Stand with your feet shoulder-width apart.
- Lower your body into a squat position as if you were sitting back into a chair.

- Hold the position at the lowest point without moving up or down, engaging your quadriceps, hamstrings, and glutes.

Wall Sit Variations:

- Lean against a wall with your feet shoulder-width apart and knees bent at a 90-degree angle.
- Hold this position, keeping your back against the wall, engaging your quads, hamstrings, and glutes.

- Variations include lifting one leg, adding pulses, or using different foot positions for varying intensity.

Calf Raises Hold:

- Stand on the edge of a step or platform with your heels hanging off.
- Push through the balls of your feet to rise onto your toes.
- Hold the raised position at the top, engaging your calf muscles.

Core

Targeting the core with isometric exercises can bring excellent results. Here are some effective ones:

Plank Variations:

Standard Plank: Support your body on your forearms and toes, maintaining a straight line from head to heels.

Side Plank: Support your body on one forearm and the side of one foot, keeping your body in a straight line from head to toe, engaging your obliques.

Plank with Leg Lift: From a standard plank position, lift one leg a few inches off the ground, engaging your core to maintain balance and stability.

Russian Twists Hold:

- Sit on the floor with your knees bent and feet lifted off the ground.
- Hold a weight or medicine ball in front of you and twist your torso from side to side without moving your legs or arms, engaging your obliques and core muscles

Hollow Body Hold:

- Lie on your back, engage your core, and lift your arms and legs off the ground.
- Maintain a hollow shape with your lower back pressed into the floor, engaging your entire core.

These exercises help engage various core muscles, enhancing stability and strength in the abdominal and oblique regions. Variations can be added to intensify or modify the challenge level.

CHAPTER TWO

Dynamic Isometric Exercises

Dynamic isometric exercises combine the static contraction of isometric exercises with dynamic movements, adding intensity and variety to workouts. Some are examples of dynamic isometric exercises:

Isometric-Plyometric Combo:

- Start with an isometric hold, such as a wall sit or squat hold.
- Follow it immediately with an explosive plyometric movement,

like a jump squat or a jump from a wall sit position.

- This combination challenges muscles by transitioning from static to explosive movements, enhancing strength and power.

Isometric Ball Throws:

- Hold a medicine ball or any weighted object at chest height.
- Press the ball against a wall or floor with maximal force for a few seconds.
- Immediately release the ball and explosively throw it against a wall

or to a partner, engaging various muscles during the isometric hold and explosive release.

Isometric Band Pulls:

Attach a resistance band to a fixed object at chest height.

Hold the band with both hands, keeping it taut.

Pull the band apart, creating tension and holding the position statically, engaging your back, shoulders, and arms.

These dynamic isometric exercises combine the benefits of both isometric and dynamic movements, challenging muscles in different ways.

Isometric Partner Exercises **Partner Wall Sit Challenge:**

- Both partners assume a wall sit position with their backs against each other.
- Holding hands or linking arms, partners press against each other, adding resistance to each other's wall sit.
- This adds an element of resistance and engagement, making the wall sit more challenging.

Dual Plank Holds:

- Partners face each other in a plank position, either on elbows or extended arms.
- Maintain the plank while gently high-fiving or tapping each other's hands.
- This adds a cooperative element while maintaining stability and engagement in the core and upper body.

Resistance Band Partner Holds:

- Using a resistance band, partners face each other and hold either end of the band.
- Create tension in the band by pulling away from each other, maintaining the position for a set duration.
- This exercise engages various muscle groups, especially the arms, shoulders, and core.

Partner isometric exercises not only challenge muscles but also add an element of interaction and cooperation, making workouts more enjoyable.

Isometric Exercises with Props and Equipment

Isometric exercises using props and equipment can intensify workouts and target specific muscle groups. Here are some examples:

Stability Ball Isometric Holds:

- Plank on a stability ball by resting your forearms on the ball and keeping your body straight.
- Hold this position, engaging your core muscles for stability and balance.

TRX Isometric Exercises:

- TRX suspension trainers can be used for isometric exercises like TRX planks or TRX chest press holds.
- In a TRX plank, place your feet in the straps and hold a plank position, engaging core and upper body muscles.

Isometric Exercises Using Resistance Bands:

Perform isometric exercises like chest press holds or bicep curls by holding resistance bands at specific angles to create tension and hold the position statically.

Advanced isometric training challenging exercises

One-Arm Isometric Push-Ups:

- Get into a push-up position and lower yourself halfway.
- Lift one hand off the ground and hold the position briefly before switching to the other hand, engaging chest and triceps muscles.

Handstand Hold Variations:

- Progress from wall-assisted handstands to freestanding handstands, holding the position for increased durations to challenge shoulder and core strength.

Human Flag Progressions:

- Progress from side plank variations to eventually holding a human flag position, gripping a vertical object and holding your body parallel to the ground, engaging upper body and core muscles intensely.

CHAPTER THREE
Isometric Yoga Poses

Downward Dog Hold:

- Engages the shoulders, core, and hamstrings.
- Hold the pose for a specific duration, focusing on alignment and breath.

Warrior Pose Variations:

- Warrior I or II engage the legs, core, and arms.
- Hold these poses statically, concentrating on muscle engagement and balance.

Boat Pose Isometric Hold:

- Engages the core and hip flexors.
- Maintain the boat pose by balancing on your sitting bones while keeping the legs lifted.

Creating a Balanced Isometric Workout

To balance an isometric workout, consider targeting various muscle groups:

Upper Body Isometric Exercises: Include plank variations, isometric push-up holds, or wall push-ups.

Lower Body Isometric Exercises: Incorporate squats holds, wall sits, or calf raises holds.

Core Isometric Exercises: Add moves like plank variations, boat pose, or hollow body holds.

Yoga-Based Isometric Poses: Integrate yoga poses like downward dog, warrior poses, or boat pose.

Sample Isometric Workout Plan

Here's a sample routine:

Warm-up: 5-10 minutes of light cardio or dynamic stretching.

Isometric Exercises: Perform 3 sets of each exercise, holding for 20-60 seconds.

- Plank variations (30 sec each)
- Squat holds (45 sec)
- Boat pose isometric hold (30 sec)
- Downward dog hold (45 sec)

Cool-down: 5-10 minutes of static stretching for all major muscle groups.

Adjusting Duration: If the suggested hold times feel too challenging, start with shorter durations (e.g., 10-15 seconds) and gradually increase as you build strength and endurance.

Increasing Intensity: To intensify the workout, consider adding more sets, increasing hold times, or incorporating more challenging variations of the exercises. For instance, you can try single-leg squats or add dynamic movements after isometric holds.

Variations: Experiment with different variations of each exercise. For example, try different plank variations like side planks, forearm planks, or elevated planks to target muscles differently.

Rest Intervals: Allow adequate rest between sets to ensure proper recovery. Start with 30-60 seconds between sets and adjust based on how you feel.

Progression: As you become more comfortable with the routine, aim to progress by gradually increasing hold times, adding more challenging exercises, or incorporating weights or resistance bands for added resistance.

Isometric training for specific goals

Isometric training for specific goals and essential safety guidelines:

Isometrics for Strength Gain:

- Isometric exercises can enhance strength by recruiting muscle fibers, improving muscle endurance, and promoting neuromuscular adaptations. Focus on holding isometric exercises at specific joint angles to target strength gains in those positions.

Isometrics for Rehabilitation:

- Isometric exercises are commonly used in rehab programs as they exert less stress on injured tissues. They help maintain muscle strength and aid in the recovery process. Consult a physical therapist for specific exercises tailored to your injury.

Isometrics for Flexibility:

- While isometrics primarily focus on strength, they can indirectly improve flexibility by increasing muscle strength in elongated positions. Incorporating isometric stretches (static stretches performed with light isometric contractions) can enhance flexibility over time.

Safety Guidelines and Tips

Safety is paramount when performing isometric exercises. Here are essential safety guidelines and tips:

Breathing Techniques during Isometric Holds:

- Maintain steady and controlled breathing throughout the holds.

- **Technique:** Inhale deeply before starting the hold, and exhale slowly during the contraction. Avoid holding your breath as it can increase blood pressure and reduce oxygen flow.

Importance of Proper Form:

- Correct form is crucial for preventing injury and maximizing effectiveness.

- **Alignment:** Focus on proper body alignment and positioning for each exercise.

- **Engagement:** Ensure the targeted muscles are engaged without compromising other parts of the body.

Avoiding Overexertion and Injury:

- Start with shorter hold times and gradually progress to longer durations or higher resistance.

- **Listening to Your Body:** Stop immediately if you feel sharp pain or discomfort beyond normal exertion.

- **Rest and Recovery:** Allow adequate rest between sets to prevent overexertion and aid in muscle recovery.

Conclusion

Isometric exercises offer numerous benefits including improved strength, endurance, joint stability, and they can be performed almost anywhere without equipment.

To incorporate isometric training into your routine long-term, mix various isometric exercises, gradually increase intensity, and ensure rest days for muscle recovery. Consider a balanced workout routine that includes dynamic and isometric exercises for overall fitness.

THE END

www.ingramcontent.com/pod-product-compliance
Lightning Source LLC
Chambersburg PA
CBHW072049230526
45479CB00009B/336